Corona Viral Fevernidheeshkp88

Traditional Indian Medicine

Big Pharma Versus Donald Trump

Vasu Jayaprasad

Lulu.com

Corona Viral Fever

Traditional Indian Medicine

Index

Viral Fever

Traditional Indian Medicine

Chapter I

Introduction

Author is a lawyer with experience in environmental health Sciences from legal experiences. Immune recovery suppression was noted in poultry by veterinary scientists studying poultry related diseases. Ammonia released from poultry droppings contaminate air and causes systemic damage to poultry weakening the immunity. The condition is termed as immuno recovery suppression killing the birds. Patients suffering organ transplant are given medicines to weaken immune system. Great sage of India in his scholarly thesis Charaka Samhitha says water pollution is worse than air pollution. When air, water, land are polluted and when star constellation is harmful even medicinal properties of plants will be lost. Natural ability of individuals with healthy habits may not protect him. Charaka understood concepts of public health. Pancha Karma treatment is five types cleansing the body to enhance immunity and maximize placebo effect.

Certain virus is termed as nostril fever manageable with steam inhalation and immunity booster nutrition. When body is weakened by polluted air, water land and body by various reasons including symptomatic medication immuno recovery suppression is the result. Even weak Viruses can attack body. This knowledge was used to market a fake science labeled as AIDS. Marketing many new products was successful. But medicines designed to address the nonexistent virus like

AIDS with antiretroviral virus tablets, proved an instant failure. Withdrawal symptoms associated psychotropic drug planted in the medicine caused havoc by inducing inflammatory response and death. Such beastly medication incited protests from public. Media hype, government funded propaganda through radio and television channels failed to impress. Many died to inflammatiory response after cyokine storm caused by AIDS medicines. The man behind that fake science is also behind corona 19 bluffs. Seven Sisters, big pharma companies failed to make any real money from their conventional business. They are behind new game of vaccines. Continuous failures turn them to conventional propaganda game of funding movies big and small budget to inject fear into minds of people. Fear alone weakens immune system. Launching mild virus as corona 19 and launched it through airports and hospitals globally and setting up health comrades everywhere to obviate counter moves to expose fake science, also failed.

In America president exposed involvement of Director General of world health organization a former communist who destroyed whole

Ethiopia hobnobbing with China, Obama, Bill Gates Clintons and deep financial lobbies swaying the state to create fear and suspend human rights People are out scoffing the propaganda and asserting that "we accept that virus is real but we are prepared to live with risk. Life is taking necessary risk of getting cancer cardiac conditions. We are not surrendering our freedom for a fake science". In India AIDS failed as RSS chief Sudarsan ridiculed that Hiv tests are faulty as anyone under treatment for 65 diseases will be tested

AIDS positive as there is accumulation of antibodies due to immune suppression.

Chicken guinea campaign also failed I'm India as it was launched in a state well entrenched with 5000 years old Ayurveda. Simple potions cured in days where as those accepted artv tablets suffered death or inflammatory response due to cyokine storms. Many suffered lifelong injuries. All desperate attempts to market antiviral AIDS medicines, as the medicines triggered Cytokine storms leading to inflammatory lungs raising the biological oxygen demand boosting pneumonia and causing shock and death.

Traditional method in pneumonia condition is to give 3to5 drops of black cumin oil in an ounce of water3 times a day. Black jeers oil is available in all western stores. Herbal coffee made of pepper, ginger, cinnamon or cyperus rotundus boiled with pan candy is mixed with honey and lemon three times a day enhances immunity and as 'viricide'. Drinking milk boiled with a tea spoon of turmeric helps increase red blood Corpuscles. Pneumonia is always a neglected case of fever unless sodium deficiency is induced by iodised salt. Common salt is banned in India and is the cause of most pneumonia cases direct impact of maladministration exposing people to vagaries of pharma and to their fake science. A survey on the number of fatalities among members of modern medical practitioners and nurses will show that most of them die or survive after serious injury from faulty treatments. Corona will not kill but faulty treatment will. Often pneumonia deaths are due to exogenous lipoid pneumonia is listed as corona death to keep fear game active. Corona is a mild virus, but propaganda incites fear. People have decided to fight and they are out on streets asserting their rights to face risks in life without surrendering their freedom. Slowly protesters are gaining momentum all over the world.

Many conspiracy theories are afloat like links of "Deep State" with their links with Bill Gates, Bill Clinton, Obama, and George Bush through their long association in Chin. Viral fever spread can be traced though airports hospitals and labs as everything looks like command to spread virus originated from a cluster of people. Pattern of propaganda unleashed all over the world betrays conspirators. Whole variety of products and new services were kept ready even before launch of virus.

Fake science

Viral does not kill anybody. Corona 19 is considered much more durable vius made in laboratory by blending ordinary corona virus with saars virus and H1N1 viruses. There are strong allegations that there is a new game of getting viral vaccine patented and patent holder influenced world leaders to grant production license to big pharma for production of vaccines. Indications are as early as October 2019 corona flu started appearing without causing harm as even sip of vodaka destroyed fatty coating of corona killing nucleic acid content. WHO made a calculated move and issued instructions that vodka or any liquor will not sterilise virus. But most liqour barons were licensed to makc sanitisers with alcohol. So WHO took care more to protect virus than people. World health organization now ridiculed as china health organization issued guidelines to lock down countries and force people to stay indoors. Scientists globally asserted lock down is not supported by scientific study. All studies show indoor life weakens resistance. Exposure to sun and humidity increases vitamin D production in the body and weaken the virus.Then how WHO guidelines supported fake science.

President of United States Obama in 2014 sanctions millions to North Carolina immune research lab Through Dr.Fauci directotor f national institute of allergy and infectious diseases center for corona virus research. The fund reaches China vius research institute with corona virus from American lab in north Carolina in 2015. Dr.Fauci announces virus pandemic hitting the whole world.Big pharma moves their research stations to Wuhan in China.Tedrus Adhanom a former comrade and director of WHO was hobnobbing with China to cover up the pandemic. Now the whole world is clamoring for resignation of Tedrus Adhanom.In USA doctors came out through social media that money is offered as high as 13,000$ per death to alter record and declare as viral patient $19.39000 per is offered to ensure that the patient dies with viral fever incredible version!

Is the virus created a fear psyche by blowing out of proportion? Scientists assert that fear psyche weakens immune system. Lock down keep people away from sunlight and vitamin d generation in body a natural process. Continued use of masks creates hypoxia oxygen deficiency weakening the immune system. World health organization is no wonder called China health organization. Funds are flowing heavily into key figures.

Global communism and capitalism is the only objective?

Judy A.Mikovits Biochemist, researcher in molecular biologist researching on viruses jailed for many years that AIDS is not caused by gays. Her study clearly states that immunity deficiency generally occurs in non vegetarians in comparison with vegetarianism. That condition manifest itself as meat poisoning in common parlance and scientific term is multiple sclerosis the root of a thousand diseases ranging from inflammatory responses to cancer. It is her study that is robbed by Dr. Anthony Fauci robbed and presented as gays disease. She revealed that her theory is that nonvegetarians have generally weak immune system. That is supported by age old pancha karma treatment 5000years ago by Indian saint in charaka samhitha.The lady suffered like Copernicus in this age. Her study outlined that virus do not kill but weak immune system and faulty medication also kills.

Medical jargons like allergy and syndrome are lavishly employed by fake science to cover up ignorance of the scientific community. Modern medicines are not able to scientifically explain or cure many ailments. Such ailments pass off as allergies. Scientist Lyall Watson in his renowned book Heavens Breath describes specialist as a person who knows more and more about less and less. In the end a specialist is a person who knows all about nothing. It is heartening to find what is painted as a global pandemic is distilling down to family pandemic affecting the families of international conmen now in firing line in USA. Armed with truth and support of virtuous men globally President of

United States is leading a war reducing global pandemic to pandemic of families of conmen. Insider information helped them to prepare well in advance for brisk business. Well-orchestrated propaganda indicates a deep association with the conspirators of virus theory. Is this just business or a bigger agenda set by league of the just? History of evangelical body international Christian league league of the just men transforming into league of the just through historical propaganda has to be probed.

Methodologies used to ban cannabis, market AIDS business, Saars Ebola is used after much more homework. It will turn out to be a great failure as network is within the reach of common man. Conspirators under estimated the power of common man. Historians will record after colossal failure of vaccine lobby behind corona virus. As common man also sees the leaders they see with thcir heart. Heart perceives truth better than brain. With failure of corona 19 pharma lobby, seven Sisters will go into bankruptcy.

Chapter II

Ayurveda

Charaka samhitha meaning charaka's code is 5000 years old medical code of acient India.Code refers to public health issues arising from contaminated air water land flora and fauna. It also refers to health issues from star constellations inducing health issues.

Ayurvedic treatment is founded on right nutrition simple medicines and purification of the body through pancha karma. Ayurvedic medicines are antiviral anti-inflammatory and neutralises Cytokene storm which causes death.

Corona being a weak virus will not survive above 30*C. Normal human temperature being 37*C corona can survive only in orifices like mouth nose and wind pipe sticking on mucus membrane. Inhalation of steam is used to kill and clear viruses in the nose and mouth.

Gargling saltwater with turmeric and edible oil is traditional life style to combat viruses everyday without waiting for symptoms of viral attack. Water is boiled with eucalyptus oil or mint with caraway seed or basal leaves and vapour is inhaled to free orifices from viral attack. When a person experiences sore throat nasal congestion this is the first precautionary step. Basil leaves is a proven antiviral anti-bacterial anti-fungal medicinal. It is worshipped as a holy plant in India. Eucalyptus and tree tea oils are antiviral. Herbal coffee made of ginger which has anti-viral property is boiled in water with cyperus rotundus a powerful antiviral rhizome. Lemon and honey is added after decanting into a cup and drinking three times a day clear viral infections. Basil leaf is antipyretic.

Panchakarma procedure is purification of body following five different detoxification processes. Body is strengthened by immunity boosting nutrients packed in medicines. All nutrition that supports illness is avoided. High protein diet is avoided in Ayurvedic treatment unlike modern systems. Herbal soup and fruits, vegetables, nuts are preferred. Pathyam means what is liked by disease.Ayurveda has a deep understanding of medicinal food and life, style disorders. They have a perfect understanding of medical properties of plants by understanding terrains and celestial position of stars. Corona cure is by, antiviral chemicals like Cyperene derived from plants used in combination with antipyretic antimicrobial herbs. Herbal soups and raw fruits and vegetables are preferred. Fifty percentage of cure in ayurveda is through nutrition.   a catalyst

Chapter III
Vulnerable to Corona.
1. Age

Aged persons and children are more vulnerable to any common flu.Young children often get 2or 3 corona infections and are considered heathy. Children develop immunity after each infection. Children are encouraged to play in mud to get such infections as part of immunity development. Such infections are natural vaccinations.

Older persons develop weak immune system due to a variety of reasons. Most common condition is acidified body due to damaged villi in the small intestine which alkalises the body.

Any virus or cancer cell gets killed when it comes into contact with an alkaline environment ranging from 7 to 14. Alkaly react with fatty covering breaking open nucleic acid. Alkaly neutralised acid content of corona. Even older people are unaffected as they traditionally follow a life style of going to bed with a peg of whisky or after gargling with saltwater mixed with edible oil. But chronic patients who are on inflammatory medicines are vulnerable to any viral fevers. Proper medicines are not normally followed in modern medicine due to ignorance or greed.

Vitamin C is recommended as antiviral and anti inflammatory by researchers. But Why WHO has not recommended vitamin C megadose. World health organisation do not recommend megadose or adequate doses for corona 19. Why? Linus C pauling was given nobel Prize for his vitamin C megadose theory. World Health organisation heavily funded by world governments is apparently hobnobbing with corona 19vaccine lobby.

Corona is not a killer. But many deaths are reported as corona mostly people in the age group of 80 and above. A doctor in US reported that there were instructions to him to report a 96 years old lady's death as corona death ostensibly to maintain a fear psyche in the mind of public. Is administration also in a conspiracy to promote corona scare. Even world health organisation published guidelines founded mostly on fake science. Global governments except US administration swallowed fake science.

World Health Organization in the guidelines categorically asserts there is no cure for viral fevers like corona 19. WHO is expected to know the existance of Antiviral medicines from their own publication or their consultant research labs like national council of biotechnology institute NCBI in US. Nobel laureate Linus C Pauline promulgated vitamin C mega dose for viral and bacterial infections. Vitamin C mega dose stops cytokine storm triggered by antibodies when corona virus colonises. In rabbies also cytokine storm causes death. As elderly people have weak cells cytokine storm instead of attacking virus triggers auto immune disorder creating a situation where immune cells start attacking weak body causing ordema. Water content in the blood stream swells triggering inflammation. RBC content in lungs gets outnumbered triggering pneumonia, shock and death.

Healthy person may not even recognise corona19 viral fever. Then why this orchestrated propaganda? Coffee is a proven hypochondrium. It clears 50% of liver fibrosis cirrhosis. Enhanced liver is the best defender. Best drink in old age is black coffee with ginger coves or cinnamon with a bit of turmeric. Such beverages three times a day enhances heart liver and kidney function. Virus doesn't kill but lowered immunity kills. Corona will not kill normal inflammatory response of the body inducing biological oxygen demand creates breathing difficulties pneumonia and death in the aged.

2. Cardiac patients

Cardiac patients who are on statin poison, analgesics or pain killers are more vulnerable to any viral fevers. Millet diet enhances RBC count. Inflammatory food such as wheat rich in gluten may be avoided. People who are lactose intolerant should boil milk with a teaspoon of turmeric to enhance RBC level. Pneumonia patients may require blood transfusion to boost RBC level. Most medicines given to heart patients are inflammatory.

3. Cancer

Chemotherapy is injecting cyanide into the body. Patient's immune system will be very weak. Mild viruses like corona 19 will have a killer impact on such patients. Cancer is not curable in conventional oncology. When infected with corona virus vitamin C mega dose is the best option. Traditional Indian medicine TCM offers cure in any disease caused by multiple sclerosis. Cure is scattered among physicians and locating right physicians need, guidance in the form of referrals. Black cumin oil is a safe medicine for cardiac, cancerous, diabetic patients. Koran recommends black cumin oil as a last resort. I have observed absolute overnight recovery for acute a pneumonia patient rocked by cytokine storm.

Chapter IV

Confronting Corona

There are many options for many simple options for viral flue treatment. Bigpharma is at big margine. Not really interested efficient cure. Their foundations may media hype. Accounts of big foundations who has links with global corona marketing is being investigated.

1. Herd immunity is the best practice. People brave the disease. Eat and dine with the

patients and celebrate disease as blessing of God. Modern pharmacopoeias also consider herd immunity as a best practice. Children getting best immunity by exchanging infections in the school are well founded scientific and healthy practice. Nature is full of microbes. Life is everyday battle. Lockdown for mild flu is height of nonsense. World health organization guidelines are fake science.

2. Gargling everyday with salt and edible oil and with a pinch of turmeric in warm water is effective anti-bacterial practice.

3. Holding a spoonful of edible oil in the mouth for a few minutes pierces fatty envelop of any virus leaving open nucleic acid of virus to be dissolved by digestive juices. Spit out the oil and saliva this is called oil pull. This practice strengthens teeth. Oil permeates teeth and ensures enhanced transportation of calcium.

4. Smearing oil in the nose and ears with edible oil is a simple defense to check viral deposits.

5 Black coffees clean up liver. Black coffee made with basil leaves, ginger, turmeric, cinnamon or cyperous rotundus (mutanga) is the best anti viral health drink. In ayurveda it is

called second kashaya meaning herbal tea. When inflected one has throat pain stuffy nose or inflammatory responses like body pain, fever. Drink the tea three times a day. Coffee is the best drink to clear fifty percentage of fibrosis in liver and lungs.Turmeric is proven antiviral rhizome. Zinc content penetrates cells and enables antiviral medicines like quinine to kill any virus.

6. Stuffy nose is an indication of accumulation and multiplication of virus in the sinus cavities. Inhale steam with eucalyptus oil. Mild viral attacks with virus which get destroyed are

termed nostril fever cleared with stem inhalation with eucalyptus oil or caraway seeds. Medicated clay rasnadi powder is burned in cotton roll and hot smoke 2000*C is inhaled to kill and clear viral clusters in sinus clusters. Cigarette tipped with cannabis leaves if smoked by pushing the fumes through nose kills virus. Cannabinoids help immune cells to neutralize and kill gramme negative bacteria and heals pneumonia.

7. Drink one ounce of doshi jeet ayurvedic decoction three times a day to trigger antiviral combat against chicken guinea SAARS, EBOLA.

Corona19 is a combination of these viruses but falls into categories of weak viruses. A rabbi also is not a killer virus only edema damages the brain and kills patient. Ayurveda has medicines to ease water pressure in the brain instantaneously.

8. Lemon juice reduces Cytokine storm. It is anti viral and will also dehydrate body reducing inflammation.

9. Intravenous application of vitamin C mega dose is the safest effective cure. It is propounded By Linus C Pauling.

10. Lypospheric C produced by Livon laboratories is an excellent antiviral soup addressing enhancing internal organs like kidney lungs heart will be enhanced .It is a powerful antioxidant vitalizing cells.

11. Blood transfusion enhances RBC content in blood reducing biological oxygen demand.

12. Black cumin oil 3 to 5 drops in one ounce of water clear accumulated water in lungs. Ensure overnight cure of pneumonia.

13. Soaking hen's egg in undiluted lemon juice for 12 hours packs eggs eye with vitamin C. Emulcified vitamin C is absorbed fully

absorbed into blood stream and acts as a powerful antiviral nutrition. Emulsified vitamin C is sold in US by Livon lab.

The present pandemonium is disguised war for economic dominance. Do not accept any guideline without checking as authorities like World health organization commands least respect. Present viral scam is a war between fake science and truth. Armed with social media and ebook let us fight this war.

Disclaimer

Author is a lawyer and has no special knowledge about viral fevers or its cure. The contents of the book are informations collected from the authors field of nleagal practice and appraisal of comparative study of medicines.Readers are cautione3d to further enhance their knowledge absolve themselves from any injury.